Real Food Diet

Easy Healthy Eating

By Cathy Wilson

Copyright © 2014

Income Disclaimer

This book contains business strategies, marketing methods and other business advice that, regardless of my own results and experience, may not produce the same results (or any results) for you. I make absolutely no guarantee, expressed or implied, that by following the advice below you will make any money or improve current profits, as there are several factors and variables that come into play regarding any given business.

Primarily, results will depend on the nature of the product or business model, the conditions of the marketplace, the experience of the individual, and situations and elements that are beyond your control.

As with any business endeavor, you assume all risk related to investment and money based on your own discretion and at your own potential expense.

Liability Disclaimer

By reading this book, you assume all risks associated with using the advice given below, with a full understanding that you, solely, are responsible for anything that may occur as a result of putting this information into action in any way, and regardless of your interpretation of the advice.

You further agree that our company cannot be held responsible in any way for the success or failure of your business as a result of the information presented in this book. It is your responsibility to conduct your own due diligence regarding the safe and successful operation of your business if you intend to apply any of our information in any way to your business operations.

Terms of Use

Real Food Diet
Easy Healthy Eating

By Cathy Wilson

Table of Contents

Introduction

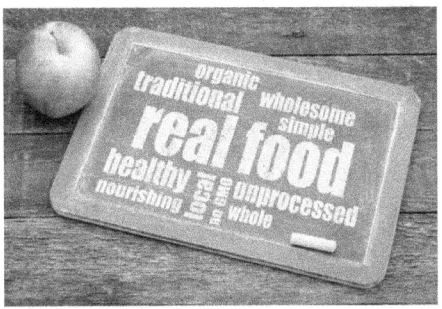

According to health experts at *The Atlantic* publication, scientists compared EVERY single diet out there, and the winner is...

REAL FOOD!

Just rewind the clock a few hundred thousand years to caveman days, and you'll notice there were no fast-food burgers, junky food corner stores, heck there wasn't even refrigeration for REAL food!

The mindset back then was totally different.

Food was an essential focus, a powerful factor of survival.

FACT: When Mother Nature wasn't on her period, food was plentiful and bellies were full. However, from time to time the hormones went a little whacky and food was scarce, resulting in environmental hardship. Natural disasters like droughts, floods or fires, could wipe out food stores instantaneously. And don't forget about deadly disease, long before conventional medicine was founded.

Times have changed...

You can say food is still a focus, but for all the wrong reasons. The last of which is nourishing your body with wholesome macronutrients, essential vitamins and minerals, and water.

COLD HARD FACT - *WE RARELY EAT BECAUSE OF PHYSIOLOGICAL HUNGER. AND IF WE DO, IT'S RARELY THE ESSENTIAL NUTRIENTS YOUR BODY CRAVES.*

According to *WebMD*, this is why we eat...

*Learned Favorite Foods

*Looks Good

*Convenience/Cost

*Personality

*Can't Decide

*Social

Funny, **NONE** of these reasons is because your body is physiologically in need of energy to function.

Time to look into what **REAL** food eating is all about. This introductory book will help you figure out where *REAL* food fits in your life!

Chapter One - What is REAL Food?

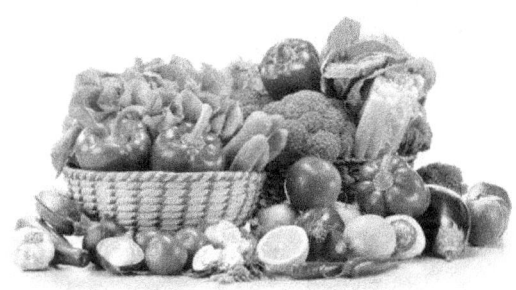

Science Daily says, your best diet is with minimally processed foods that are close to nature, focused on plants, and that help promote good health and disease prevention.

REAL FOOD is any food that's void of processing.

"Real Food Feeds and Nourishes You"

Real Food Facts:

*Food in its natural state, which is unprocessed, or has very little processing.

*Doesn't need snazzy packaging or labelling.

*Real Food is a natural whole food that sustains life.

*Nothing is taken away.

*Food eaten in its natural state.

*Whole grains where the whole grain is milled, not parts of it.

*Your body was designed to process REAL WHOLE FOODS.

Sample Real Foods

Fresh whole fruit
Veggies in their natural state - carrots, broccoli, parsnip, beans, peas, peppers, etc.
Organic meats - lower fat cuts preferred
Free-range eggs
Whole grain bread
Hard cheese
Skim milk
All-natural yogurt
Raw nuts/seeds
Steel cut oats
Quinoa
Amaranth

To help better explain REAL food, we're going to also have a look at processed or "fake" food.

PROCESSED FOOD - Has been altered from their natural state, for safety reasons, or better storage, according to abouthealth.com.

We are programmed to think all processed foods are bad. The truth is, a lot are, but not ALL of them!

Processing Methods:

*Refrigeration
*Canning
*Freezing
*Aseptic processing
*Dehydration

NOTE - It's not the method of processing that really makes many processed foods unhealthy, it's what's added during the process.

BOTTOM LINE - There are processed foods made with healthy ingredients that are okay to eat. It's the ones with added salt, fat, and sugars, or that have few nutrients, that you want to avoid.

Sample Healthy Processed Foods

*Frozen veggies
*Frozen fruit with no additives
*Low-fat milk
*Breakfast cereals made with 100% natural whole grains (watch for added sugar)
*Canned tuna in water - low sodium
*Frozen fish
*Dried fruits
*Roasted nuts/seeds

Unhealthy Processed Foods are high in saturated Trans fat, have lots of sodium and sugar, and little nutritional value. Setting you up for enlarging your waistline and negatively affecting your health.

Sample Bad Processed Foods to Avoid for the Most Part

*Breaded frozen fish sticks
*Breaded frozen chicken or chicken wings
*Canned foods like ravioli, spaghetti or macaroni, with additives
*Noodles in a cup or package
*Potatoes in a box
*Pasta made with refined white flour
*Muffin, cookie, and cake mixes where you just add water
*Snack foods like chips, crackers, candies, and packaged pastries
*Frozen dinners
*Energy drinks
*Shelf pizza mix, Hamburger Helper, and other box dinners
*Sugary breakfast cereals and packaged lunch snacks
*Soda
*Fruit drinks

*Hash browns
*Bacon, sausage, and deli meats
*Hotdogs
*Hamburg and hotdog buns
*White bread, pitas, wraps, and English muffins
*Instant pudding and jello mixes
*Energy bars
*Energy drinks
*Ice-cream
*High sugar and high salt condiments, like ketchup and barbe-
cue sauce
*Mayonnaise and dressing

Science behind Eating REAL Food

There are 5 main brain chemicals that influence what you eat, when, and how much...

Serotonin - This chemical leaves you feeling good.

Norepinephrine - Your adrenaline, or *fight* or *flight* response.

Nitric Oxide -This calms you. It helps relax your blood vessels.

Dopamine - Acts as a pain reliever. A pleasure and reward neurotransmitter.

GABA - Works like an anesthesia. Leaves you feeling like you're zoned out.

It's the combination of chemicals in your body that determines whether you're going to pig out on ice-cream, or have a single serving of low-fat yogurt. It all starts with your serotonin signaling to your brain to feel fantabulous. Your brain then breaks down the serotonin, which removes this awesome feeling.

Naturally many of us learn to reach for the junky quick high fat food, that's going to quickly make us feel fab again. Sugary food loaded with bad carbs does the trick.

The actual low from the chemical depression can trigger cravings for more unhealthy fuel, according to experts at *Your Beauty and Nutrition.*

SOLUTION - By understanding how your brain works, you can better diffuse your quick unhealthy cravings, and opt for healthy REAL foods that'll keep your blood sugars level, and give you that feel-good feeling long-term.

My Thoughts...

Real food eating is just getting back with nature. And by consciously choosing to ditch the processed crap and go for the all-natural wholesome foods, you're going to move one step closer to losing fat and getting back to the healthier, happier, smaller you!

Excuses will get you nowhere fast.

COMMIT to opening your mind to change, and it WILL happen!

Chapter Two - Benefits of Eating REAL Food

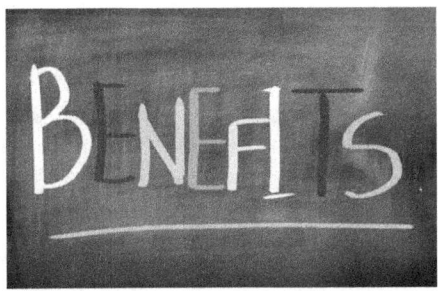

We create most of our health issues by not paying attention to what our body needs and delivering. Medical experts tell us we need to exercise, cut out fatty processed foods, make healthier lifestyle choices, and pay attention to our internal body cues.

THE TRUTH: Most of us don't. That's why we aren't as healthy as we could be.

Choosing to consume nutrient dense whole foods instead of nutrient-less processed fast foods, is your first step toward improving energy, blasting fat, deterring serious disease from implanting in you, and reducing chronic conditions that flip your switch to negative.

According to *WebMD*, scientists have uncovered hundreds of biologically active plant-food components called phytonutrients. These are naturally protective antioxidants that shield your body from disease, and boost your immune system function.

The Point... Flood your body with natural plant foods and you will strengthen your immune system function.

BONUS - Scientists believe there are oodles more of these protective nutrient chemicals to be found. And the only way you're going to find them, is to eat a wide variety of healthy REAL food.

Real Food Benefits Include...

*Naturally Occurring Vitamins and Minerals to Strengthen and Nourish Your Body

Science shows natural foods are more easily absorbed and utilized than supplements. Which are chemical structures that try to get close to natural for optimal body gain. But they aren't the real deal.

*No Extra Sugar

Sugar just gets you into trouble. With natural foods you don't have to worry about added sugars. Sure, there are some natural sugars, particularly in fruits, but your body is built to handle that.

Processed sugars and white sugars trigger fat storage, depression, and anxiety. They're also linked to diabetes, cardiovascular disease, poor immune system function, and cavities.

*No Bad Addictions

Sugars, additives, and preservatives are addictive. So if you chomp down one cookie, there's an increased chance you'll want more and more. With **REAL** food you don't **O.D.** on sugar. This means you're not likely to let emotions take control and urge you to overeat.

According to *LiveScience,* some junk food is as addictive as drugs!

*Smart Carbs

Natural foods give you the carb energy you need without all the issues simple sugar carbohydrates do. Avoiding the unhealthy sugars you get eating pastries and cakes. Which shoot your blood glucose levels through the roof for short periods of time, and then zap your energy just as quickly. Both of which are very unhealthy.

*No Surprise Fat

In processed foods the fat is often hidden. So even when you *think* something is healthy or fat-free off the shelf, the ingredient list may indicate otherwise.

Processed foods often have "bad" fat, or saturated Trans fat. These fats increase the risk of heart disease, diabetes, stroke, Alzheimer's, and obesity.

REAL food has fat, but it's "good" fat, or unsaturated. For instance, nuts are extremely healthy, but in moderation. One serving is just an ounce of mixed nuts. That's about 20 average size nuts. Giving you about 160 calories, 6 grams of protein, and 14 grams of total fat. Take note, one serving delivers about 35% of vitamin E, and 30 % of manganese, according to *Livestrong.*

So just don't get caught waiting for a seat in the restaurant, sipping a beer at the bar and munching on nuts! That's going overboard with the healthy.

*No Worries with the Salt

Overloading your body with salt stresses out your kidneys and boosts blood pressure.

REALITY - Too much salt ends up as just another toxin your body has to try and get rid of.

Minimal sodium is essential to good health. According to *The Naked Scientist,* you need salt to help regulate cell function. From electrical impulses, to calcium absorption, salt is required.

Processed or unnatural food has oodles of salt. This increases your intrinsic desire to have more, stressing your system.

*You Know What's Going In Your Body

Sugar, salt, added fat and preservatives, are downright dangerous. When you eat healthy whole foods, you eliminate the guess work. You know you're putting the best possible nutrition into your body. And no matter what you choose or how much. It's better than processed unhealthy crap any day of the week!

CDC, or Center for Disease Control and Prevention, reports more than seventy-five percent of sodium consumed by Americans comes from processed fast food.

Something to think about!

*Fiber is REAL!

Unfortunately many processed foods are packaged pretty, and make misleading claims about the nutrient value inside. Bran muffins are called healthy, even if they've only got 5% REAL bran! The rest can be synthetic and over-processed wheat, which of course has been stripped of essential vitamins and minerals. So you're getting a nice big wallop of fat with very little fiber, and no nutrition, in your supposedly healthy bran muffin.

Just because a product says it has fiber, doesn't mean the quantity is significant or healthy.

Getting your fiber from natural whole grains, beans, nuts, fruits and veggies, minus the processing, is your best route to healthy!

Here are a few more benefits of healthy whole food eating...

- *Better brain function*
- *You'll be happier*
- *Better control of your weight*
- *You'll have the tools to handle stress better*
- *You will eat less because your body will register full*
- *You won't look your age*
- *Your health will be better*
- *You will spend less money overall*
- *You'll live longer than your processed food friends*

My Thoughts...

You are what you eat is true. If you choose to eat unhealthy refined and processed foods, you're gambling with your health. Unnatural means your body doesn't quite know what to do with it. These processed foods are seen as "toxic," and often end up stuck in the cells of your body because your system doesn't have the ability to get rid of them.

Over time, this manifests into disease that can't be reversed.

*You best step is to take action today. Make the changes that are going to fill your body full of **REAL** food, and reap the rewards of good health!*

Chapter Three - Nutrition Your Body Needs

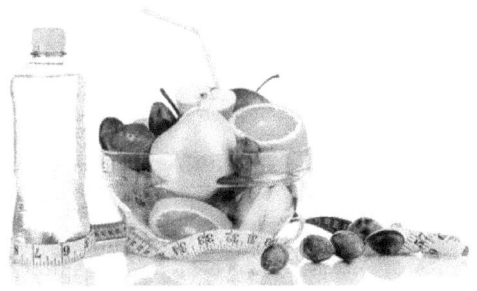

What are Essential Nutrients?

Essential nutrients are nutrients your body can't make, or at least not enough of it, according to experts at *Healthy Eating*. This means you have to find these nutrients in the foods you eat.

In order for your body to function optimally you need SIX essential nutrients; carbohydrates, protein, fat, minerals, vitamins, and water.

Carbs, protein, and fat are macronutrients. Your body needs them in large amounts.

Vitamins and Minerals are classified as micronutrients, because your body requires them in smaller quantities.

Carbohydrates

Fact: Carbs are the main source of energy for your brain. If you didn't get any carbs, you'd have a tough time functioning at all for long.

Carbohydrate Sources:

*Healthy whole grains

*Fruits and starchy veggies

*Sugars (natural)

Benefits of Whole Grains and Fruits - You get oodles of fiber, which helps remove toxic waste, reduce the risk of heart disease, and stabilize blood glucose levels.

There are TWO types of carbohydrates; complex and simple; good and bad.

Complex Carbohydrates - Provide longer lasting energy because they take longer to break down. These carbs tend to have a nice dose of fiber, which also gives you that full feeling after eating.

Good Carb Examples - Are whole grains like whole grain pasta and rice, whole wheat bread, rye, barley, oats, buckwheat, and whole grain corn.

Specifically, whole grains are loaded with protective phytochemicals, fiber, and vitamins and minerals critical to great health. They're also good for your blood glucose levels, because these carbs help keep them steady, with slow release energy.

Fruits, veggies, and legumes are also examples, because they're chalk full of a diverse range of nutrients that are often low-fat, high fiber, and plentiful in carbs and protein.

Simple Carbohydrates - Give your body short term energy gain. They also spike blood glucose levels, which is linked to diabetes.

Depression, obesity, and mood swings are associated with simple sugar carbs. You can find them naturally in fruits and milk products, along with sugars, that are added through processing. Cakes, pastries, and white pasta are loaded with white flour and added sugars, making them "bad" carb choices.

Bad Carb Examples - White bread, pretzels, pizza crust, muffins, biscuits, donuts, and hotdog buns, are all examples simple carbs with little nutritional value, and short-term energy.

What Happens?

During the processing, these foods are refined. Where they're beat to death and stripped of all their essential vitamins and minerals. Add to that, the fact they have typically high glycemic index numbers, which means they'll trigger chaos with your blood sugar levels.

More Examples...

-Soda
-Crackers
-Chips
-Sweets
-Cookies
-Pancakes
-Pastries
-Baked goods

CIP - Cathy's Important Point - Research studies from the *University of Waterloo*, found simple carbs trigger a blood sugar level drop, which affects the part of your brain linked to impulse control. Experts conclude this leads to a loss of self-control. Which of course triggers unhealthy emotional eating, habitual eating, obesity, and increased disease and illness.

Smart Move

Nutritionists from *Canadian Living* suggest approximately 250 grams of good carbs for the average 1800 calories/day regimen. This equates to up to 65 percent of your total nutrient intake.

FACT: Carbs technically aren't critical to your survival, cuz your system has the ability to get fuel from protein and fat. However, that's not usually an idea. Cuz then you're playing around with ketones. This can easily get out of hand with dire consequences, under extreme circumstance.

It's a choice. Taking out complex carbs will also reduce your food selection substantially, and increase the odds you're going to be vitamin deficient.

Low carb diets are typically great for weight loss, but so are smart low-fat balanced **REAL** food eating.

Protein

Protein is the building block of life. Every single cell in your body has protein, according to health and wellness guru *Dr. Oz*!

Protein helps build muscle and maintain and repair cell tissue. If you break protein down, you'll have 20 amino acids. All of which are necessary for a complete protein.

More Protein Facts...

*Of these 20 amino acids, 9 are essential and must be provided thought diet

*Up to thirty-five percent of your daily energy should come from lean protein sources.

What's a complete protein?

This food source has all 20 amino acids present for optimal health. For the most part, these complete proteins are from animal sources.

Complete Protein Sources...

*Turkey and chicken
*Meat
*Milk and milk products
*Eggs
*Fish

Experts at *Fitday*, say if even one essential amino acid is missing, the protein is not complete!

What's an incomplete protein?

It's a protein source that doesn't have all 20 pieces of the puzzle. Or at least not in the appropriate amounts. Often incomplete proteins are plant sources. So it is possible to get complete proteins through vegan eating. But you'll have to mix and match your sources just like putting a puzzle together, in order to get useable complete proteins.

Incomplete Protein Sources...

*Beans
*Nuts and seeds
*Grains

*Peas and corn

Benefits of Protein:

*Greater muscle mass and lean tissue - Protein helps boost your metabolism and energy so that lean muscle is gained and fat is lost.

*Keeps nails, hair and skin healthy

*Lower calorie intake and less hunger - According to *Men's Fitness*, diets high in protein are known to zap fat. Protein fills you up with long lasting energy. This makes you feel full longer. So naturally you eat less to feel satisfied.

*Less risk of osteoporosis - Studies show that adequate protein intake improves bone density and lowers the risk of bone breakdown.

*Improved thinking - High protein food helps promote energy, wakefulness, motivation, and optimal thought function. The nutrients in protein make your brain work better!

*Improved sleep - Protein seems to have the intrinsic chemical message to tell your body when it should be sleeping and when it's awake time. Scientists report healthy protein eating promotes a restful night's sleep.

*Decreases blood pressure - According to *Poliquingroup*, higher levels of protein in the diet lowers blood pressure significantly in individuals suffering from hypertension.

*Injury recovery faster - With increased protein synthesis you increase the speed of tissue repair. And having stronger tendons and muscles because of eating protein decreases your risk of injury.

*Improved quality of life and length - By choosing to fuel your body the way nature intended, with **REAL** food and optimal complete protein, you're going to increase your overall quality of life, and the time you get to enjoy it.

EMERGENCY NOTE - People that go overboard with the protein and don't get enough healthy carbs may enter a state of ketosis. This is where your body starts burning fat for fuel instead of readily available glucose. The product of broken down fat are ketones, which are released into your blood stream for energy. In extreme situations ketones can reach dangerous levels.

Ammonia may build up in your system, and to date, experts don't know the long-term consequences of this.

There's also the concern of lack of calcium absorption with too much protein.

It's advised that you're followed by a medical practitioner when tinkering with extreme high protein and low-carb eating to lose weight.

FANTABULOUS NEWS! None of this is cause for concern if you're focusing on healthy **REAL** food eating and looking to get your normal 2-3 servings of protein per day!

NOTE - According to the US Department of Health and Human Services, the average adult needs about 2-3 servings per day of protein, totaling about 5-6 ounces. Or 45 grams per day for women, and 56 grams per day for men.

What happens if you don't get your protein?

Most people don't have to worry here, cuz we are a meat hungry society. But if you happen to be vegetarian, or dieting in the extreme, you'll want to watch out for these signs you're not getting enough protein in your diet.

SYMPTOMS OF PROTEIN DEFICIENCY

*Losing muscle
*Extreme fatigue
*Increase in illness
*More injuries
*Slow healing
*More infections
*Confusion
*Trouble concentrating
*Dizziness or fainting

Livestrong experts remind us protein deficiency is a serious issue. A breakdown of your body from the inside out.

Fat

Without fat you wouldn't exist. *Mercola* states your brain is comprised of about 60% fat. It gives you energy and helps transform fat-soluble vitamins to an absorbable form. This includes vitamins K, D, E, and A.

Experts suggest up to 35% of you daily calories should come from healthy fat sources. Including omega-3 rich foods like salmon, nuts, and olive oil.

NOTE: For the most part you don't have to fret over getting enough fat. What's important is minimizing the healthy fat in your diet, and avoiding the bad fat altogether.

2-3 tablespoons of fat is all you need per day to stay healthy!

*According to *Mayoclinic,* it's the type and amount of fatty acid in foods that dictates how fat will affect your health.

There are two main fat groups for our purpose; saturated bad fat, and unsaturated healthy fat.

Unsaturated Healthy Fat - The *National Heart Foundation* states your diet should include healthier monounsaturated and polyunsaturated fats.

MONOUNSATURATED FAT - Is found in peanuts, plant-based cooking oils, seeds, almonds, cashews, walnuts, olives, and avocado.

Serving Size Newsflash - Remember just 1-2 tablespoons of oil, or 1/4 cup of nuts is a serving.

POLYUNSATURATED FAT - These are omega-6 fats that are essential to healthy brain function. You'll find them in fatty fish like salmon and tuna, along with sesame seeds, sunflower seeds, and Brazil nuts!

National Heart Foundation recommends you get 2-3 servings of oily fish each week for optimal heart health protection.

Benefits of Healthy Fats:

*Increases HDL (good) cholesterol
*Lower risk of heart disease
*Boosts long-term energy
*Assists in fat-soluble vitamin absorption
*Protects organs
*Provides structure for cells
*Ensures optimal brain function

Good Fat Food Sources...

*Olive and olive oil
*Avocado
*Sesame oil
*Sunflower oil
*Almond oil
*Peanut butter
*Nuts and seeds
*Fatty omega-rich fish like salmon and tuna
*Tofu
*Soymilk
*Walnuts

Saturated Bad Fat; Saturated and Trans

Saturated Fat - Comes mostly from animal sources and full-fat dairy. It raises LDL or bad cholesterol, increases your risk of heart disease, diabetes, numerous cancers, and obesity.

Trans Fat - There is some minute traces of trans fat in animal products. But if you're eating the recommended 2-3 servings per day, you've got nothing to worry about. In fact, some research states small amounts of natural animal trans fat can be protective.

Problem is, most trans fat is synthetic, and created from partially hydrogenated oil. Which science says increases cholesterol levels and boosts your risk of cardiovascular disease and stroke. Cookies, cakes, pastries, fried fast food, packaged crackers, chips, and sweets, often have these dangerous synthetic trans fats.

Bad Fat Food Sources...

*Candy bars

*Margarine
*Crackers
*Muffins
*Popcorn
*Chips
*Donuts
*Pastries
*Cakes
*Cookies
*Pizza dough
*Fried fast food
*Lard
*Full-fat ice cream
*Full-fat dairy products
*Butter
*Cheese
*Poultry skin
*High fat cuts meat

NOTE: Coconut oil is an exception to the rule here. It's a saturated (bad) fat technically, solid at room temperature, but in moderation it is fantastic for your health!

Consequences of Bad Fat

Moderation is the key in everything. And too much of anything isn't good.

If you opt to load up with too many bad fat foods, here are a few of the consequences you may face:

*Increased risk for heart disease and stroke
*Plaque buildup in arteries
*Low energy
*Less oxygen available to organs
*Increased risk of cancer
*Decreased mobility and motility

*Higher risk of obesity
*Shorter lifespan
*Decreased quality of life
*Increased risk of diabetes and a whole whack of other serious diseases

Vitamins and Minerals

Vitamins and minerals are essential to good health in small amounts. By eating a healthy diverse and balanced REAL food diet, you should get all the vitamins your body needs. Unless of course you've got an underlying health condition, in which you'll need to see your doctor to create an action plan.

Vitamin C is important for the synthesis of collagen, providing structure to bones, ligaments and blood vessels. Bright veggies, citrus fruits, and berries, are typically high in this vitamin. Vitamin D aids with the absorption of vitamin C. There are numerous foods like milk and cereals that are fortified with vitamin D to help attain optimal health.

Here are some of the vitamins and minerals you need to stay healthy!

Calcium - 1000 - 1200 mg daily - found in dairy, yogurt, hard cheese, fortified cereals, and kale.

Purpose - Aids in bone growth, muscle contraction, and blood clotting.

Copper - 900 - 1000 mg daily - found in bran cereal, whole grains, seeds, nuts, and seafood.

Purpose - Aids in iron processing.

Fiber - 20-30 grams per day - found in oatmeal, peas, lentils, fruits, and veggies.

Purpose - Rids your body of harmful free-radical toxins, levels blood sugars, and makes you feel full!

Folate - 400 - 400 micrograms per day - found in whole grains, leafy greens, and fortified cereals.

Purpose - Essential for heart health, cell development, and fetal development.

Iron - 8 - 10 mg per day - found in beans, leafy greens, and turkey, beef, eggs, spinach, and soy beans.

Purpose - Optimal red blood cell and enzyme function.

Manganese - 2-3 mg per day - found in legumes, tea, whole grains, and nuts.

Purpose - Aids in enzyme formation and bone health.

Potassium - 4700 mg per day - found in milk, tuna, yogurt, and potatoes.

Purpose - Decreases risk of kidney stones, and levels blood pressure.

Sodium - Maximum 1500 mg per day - added to food.

Purpose - Balances internal fluid.

Vitamin B1 or Thiamine - 1 mg per day - found in fortified whole grain foods.

Purpose - Aids in carbohydrate and protein processing.

Vitamin B6 - 1.3 mg per day - found in chickpeas, organ meats, and fortified cereals.

Purpose - Important for infant brain development, metabolism and immune system function.

Vitamin C - 75 - 100 mg per day - found in bright veggies, citrus fruits, berries, broccoli, and tomatoes.

Purpose - Aids in collagen production, immune system function, and helps prevent cell damage from free radicals.

Zinc - 8 - 10 mg per day - found in fortified cereals, seafood and red meat.

Purpose - Important for reproduction and nerve system regulation.

FULL LIST

*Calcium
*Choline
*Chromium
*Copper
*Fiber
*Fluoride
*Folic Acid
*Iodine
*Iron
*Magnesium
*Manganese
*Molybdenum
*Phosphorus
*Potassium
*Selenium
*Sodium
*Vitamin A
*Thiamine
*Riboflavin

*Niacin
*Pantothenic Acid
*Vitamin B6
*Biotin
*Vitamin B12
*Vitamin C
*Vitamin D
*Vitamin E
*Vitamin K
*Zinc

Water

If you didn't drink water, you wouldn't be alive. Water helps transports vital nutrients to your cells, and ensures balance within your body. It removes waste from your body, and provides energy.

Healthy Eating suggests a minimum of 2-3 liters per day.

Benefits of Water...

Boosts Energy - Fights Fatigue - Your brain is about 60% water. So it makes sense that water helps you think clearly, focus and concentrate better, and boosts energy levels.

Rids Body of Toxins - Drinking lots of water helps your body get rid of harmful free-radical build up, reduces kidney stones, and the chance of getting a bladder infection.

Aids in Weight Loss - Water fills you up so you're less likely to overeat, gets rid of the by-products of fat, and boosts your metabolism. This of course helps you blast fat faster!

Reduces Headaches and Migraines - Dehydration is often a trigger for head pain. Drinking oodles of water is a great preventative move.

Improves Immune System Function - Studies show people that drink adequate amounts of water are less likely to suffer from illness in general.

Improves Skin - Water cleans out your body, which of course helps smooth out your complexion. Water also fills your cells and reduces the look of wrinkles.

Reduces Muscle Cramping - Water hydrates your body, so muscle cramps or spasms are less likely to occur.

Consequences of Water Deficiency...

Dehydration - When your body doesn't get enough water to function normally, it's called dehydration. With mild dehydration you can recover easily by drinking some water. You may be dehydrated if you're feeling thirsty, tired, dizzy, have a headache, are constipated, or you're not peeing like you should.

THE DANGER ZONE - SEVERE HYDRATION - This is where you need to seek immediate medical attention. Symptoms are heart palpitations, severe thirst, no sweating, dry mouth, sunken eyes, and little to no peeing.

Seizures - Your internal electrical circuitry is extremely critical to optimal body function. Dehydration interferes with the electrical signals between your brain and body, which can screw up your heart function, and muscle contractions. This may trigger seizures and unconsciousness. If left unattended, it can even result in death.

Heat Exhaustion - It's your hypothalamus that directs your body temperature, thirst, and hunger. If you don't have enough water in your body, when you get hot your hypothalamus has no water to release to cool you down. Trapped heat builds and results in extreme fatigue, headache, nausea, dizziness, heart palpitations, extreme thirst, and clammy skin.

If left unattended, heat exhaustion can progress to heat stroke, which inevitably can eventually lead to a heart attack, stroke, or coma in severe cases, according to experts at *Healthy Living*.

Hypovolemic Shock - Low blood volume is the main symptom of hypovolemic shock. Without adequate amounts of water in your body, your heart can't pump enough oxygen and vital nutrients to all your organs. This condition is life-threatening if not treated immediately.

Symptoms are disorientation, extreme weakness, sweating, clammy skin, little or no peeing, and pale skin.

Drink your 6-8 glasses of water every day and you shouldn't have anything to worry about. Getting into the habit of carrying a water bottle with you is a great way to remind yourself to drink up!

My Thoughts...

Without all the essential macronutrients, vitamins, minerals, and water your body requires, you'll have a tough time setting yourself up for optimal health. Each of these nutrients plays an important role in promoting good health.

*A wise-owl move is to eat a wide variety of healthy **REAL** foods daily. Providing your body with the fuel it needs to serve you happily for many years to come.*

Chapter Four - REAL Protein Foods

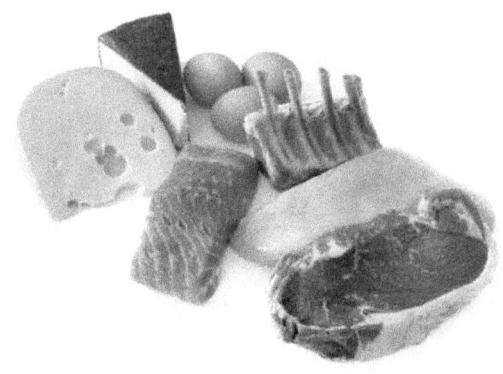

By REAL protein foods I'm referring to all-natural wholesome protein. Foods that for the most part are unprocessed and close to their natural state, void of added sugars, fats, sodium, and preservatives. A healthy REAL food diet including protein, helps blast fat and keep you healthy strong!

Healthy Living experts recommend 2-3 servings per day for a normal healthy person.

Note: You're looking to find your balance. Some high protein foods are also high in fat, so be careful.

Here's a list of optimal protein foods...

Chicken/Turkey (skinless) - 4 ounce serving, 30 grams protein, 4 grams fat

Salmon - 4 ounce serving, 20 grams protein, 7 grams fat

Tuna - 4 ounce serving, 80 calories, 20 grams protein, no fat

Top Round Steak - 4 ounces, 260 calories, 40 grams protein, 3.5 grams fat

Pork Tenderloin - 4 ounces, 110 calories, 20 grams protein, 1.5 grams fat

Bison - 4 ounces, 170 calories, 24 grams protein, 4 grams fat

Steel Cut Oats (cooked) - 3/4 cup, 125 calories, 5 grams protein, 2 grams fat

Quinoa (cooked) - 1/3 cup, 105 calories, 3.5 grams protein, 1.5 grams fat

Cooked Wild Rice - 1/3 cup, 80 calories, 2.5 grams protein, .5 grams fat

Whole Grain Bread - 1 slice, 80 calories, 3.7 grams protein, .5 grams fat

Cooked Kidney Beans - 1/3 cup, 100 calories, 7 grams protein, .3 grams fat

Lentils (cooked) - 1/3 cup, 100 calories, 7.5 grams protein, .2 grams fat

Egg - 70 calories - 6.5 grams protein, 5 grams fat

1% Milk - 1 cup, 110 calories, 6 grams protein, 4.5 grams fat

Low-Fat Yogurt - 3/4 cup, 135 calories, 10 grams protein, 3 grams fat

Sometimes it's not so easy to get your protein. I don't suggest keeping a chicken breast in your purse, of a hunk of beef in your work drawer! Here are a few protein snacks that make eating REAL protein easy!

Quick Protein Snacks

Beef Jerky - It's low-fat, and comes in oodles of protein. Just opt for the low-salt version. Jerky sports about a hundred calories an ounce.

Soy Nuts - Roasted - This changes it up from your usual nut mixture. You'll get about 8 grams of protein per 1/3 cup, and around 140 calories.

All-Natural Peanut Butter - These come in little 1.5 ounce packets, with 8 grams of protein and about 80 calories.

Hard Boiled Eggs - Two eggs is just 150 calories, and 13 grams of protein. Not to mention vitamin E, and heart healthy omega-3s.

1% Milk - One cup is just 110 calories, and delivers 6 grams of protein.

Sushi - California Rolls - Three pieces has just 100 calories, 4 grams of protein, and almost no fat.

Sashimi - Salmon - Three pieces has 100 calories, and 19 grams of protein!

Cottage Cheese - One 5 ounce serving has about 120 calories and 20 grams of protein. Just watch the salt.

Edamame - Half a cup has 8 grams of protein and less than 100 calories.

*Roasted Chickpeas - One quarter cup has 7 grams of protein and just 120 calories.

My Thoughts...

Protein is something you need to eat every day, because your body don't provide it. When you pick your protein, make sure you are sticking close with Mother Nature. Unprocessed is best, naked and not overcooked is preferable. If you plan and organize your meals, it's really quite easy to give your body the muscle-building protein it deserves!

Chapter Five - REAL Carbohydrate Foods

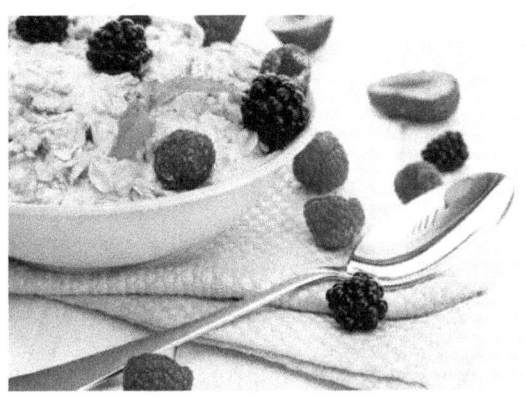

REAL carbs refers to healthy complex carbohydrates, or natural simple carbs, like fruits. It does NOT include all the processed crap you see in vending machines, boxes of the shelf, and devilish sweets and baked goods, with oodles of added sugars and fats, and crap white flour!

WebMD recommends up to 65% of your daily calories should come from carbohydrate food sources. Add to that at least 25 grams of fiber, which is often plentiful in carb foods.

Here are a few optimal REAL CARBOHYDRATE FOODS...

White Beans - 1/3 cup, 3.8 grams carbs

Barley - 1/3 cup cooked, 22 grams carbs, 75 calories, 2 grams fiber

Green Peas - 1/3 cup cooked, 50 calories, 10 grams carbs, 3 grams fiber

Whole Grain Pasta - 3/4 cup, 110 calories, 30 grams carbs, 3 grams fiber

Whole Grain Bread (whole wheat kernel) - 1 slice, 100 calories, 15 grams carbs, 3.5 grams fiber

Black Beans - 1/3 cup, 90 calories, 15 grams carbs, 6 grams fiber

Whole Oatmeal - 3/4 cup cooked, 150 calories, 25 grams carbs, 3 grams fiber

Quinoa - 1/3 cup cooked, 100 calories, 18 grams carbs, 2 grams fiber

Figs - One large, 45 calories, 10 grams carbs, 2 grams fiber

Blueberries - 1/2 cup, 40 calories, 9 grams carbs, 2 grams fiber

Quick Carbohydrate Snacks

Banana - One banana has about 80 calories and 30 grams of carbs, according to *Running Competitor.*

Brown Rice with Beans - Half a cup of rice has just 70 calories and about 20 grams of carbs. Add to that a sprinkle of steamed high-carb, fiber rich beans, and you've got one nice dose of REAL carbs!

*Low-Fat Yogurt - Many yogurts have unnecessary sugar added. Make sure you get some without added sugar. Half a cup has about 20 grams of carbs and just 50 calories. Better yet, toss in some fresh berries and you up the carbs and fiber.

Whole Grain Bread - One slice of all-natural whole grain bread has about 10 grams of carbs, and just 75 calories. Add a tablespoon of peanut better to that, and you've got complete protein for a fabulous pre-workout snack!

Whole Wheat Pasta - 3/4 of a cup has about 30 grams of carbs and just 150 calories. Add a splash of tomato sauce, and you've got some protective antioxidants to make you stronger.

Energy Bar Note - In a pinch there are all-natural energy bars you can get from your local health food store, that'll give you a good dose of carbs. Just be careful you read the ingredients. Many are loaded with extra sugars, and that's not what you're looking for.

REAL doesn't have added sugars!

My Thoughts...

Carbs are tough to transform. Particularly if you're used to eating oodles of conveniently processed simple carbohydrates with high sugar and little nutrition. It's all about taking one step at a time toward healthier REAL food eating. Try subbing one piece of your comfort white toast for a slice of whole grain. Then swap the butter for a thin layer of peanut butter. Step by step you will train your taste buds to crave wholesome goodness, minus the toxic crap additives.

Chapter Six - REAL Fat Foods

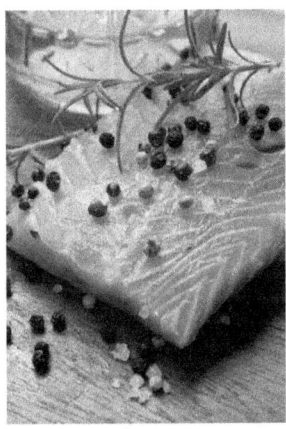

REAL Fat Foods are the same as "good" fat or unsaturated food choices, necessary for great health. To recap, they help lower bad LDL cholesterol, and boost HDL or good cholesterol. Healthy fat also provides your body with energy. It's a macronutrient your body needs for a multitude of bodily functions!

Short List - REAL Fat Foods

*Coconut Oil - 1 - 2 tablespoons, increases good cholesterol, and helps with smooth intestinal function!

*Avocado - 1/4 fruit per serving, prevents heart disease, improves memory, and is loaded with protective antioxidants.

*Salmon - 4 ounce serving, loaded with healthy omega-3s, protects the heart and wards off cancer.

*Walnuts - 5-6 pieces, loaded with protective omega 3s, anti-inflammatory properties, lowers bad cholesterol, and are chalk full of essential vitamins and minerals.

*Olive Oil - 1- 2 tablespoons, full of healthy fats, with lots of vitamin A, E, and magnesium, which helps lower cholesterol, and reduce the risk of heart disease.

Healthy Fat Note: The idea is to eat fat in moderation. By eating a healthy **REAL** food diet, you'll give your body the fat it needs to function optimally, without stepping overboard. For most people, the focus is on reducing total fat intake, not making sure they get enough.

Eat the "right" kind of fat and you're doing great!

My Thoughts...

REAL fats are healthy fats. This means staying away from fried fast foods, processed and packaged items, and making sure you stick to foods that are truly natural. You don't have to worry about getting enough good fat in your diet if you're eating a diverse range of healthy REAL foods each day. Just concentrate now on getting rid of the saturated trans fat food sources, and replacing them with the heart-healthy unsaturated ones.

Chapter Seven - Better REAL Food Choices

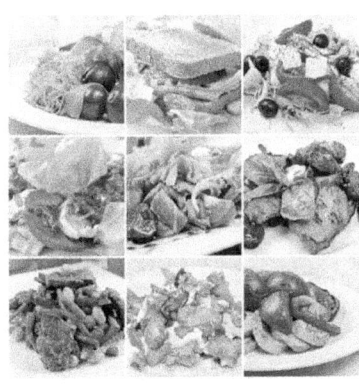

We are a society that sensationalizes food. It's our focus because we make it the center of attention. From social gatherings and work meetings, to combatting boredom and emotional stresses, we use and abuse food.

By taking the time to understand why your body needs fuel, and more specifically what type of essential nutrients it requires and in what amounts, you'll have the tools you need to reach your optimal health level.

To make it easy, I'm going to divide this next chapter into meal categories; breakfast, lunch, dinner, and snacks. This way you can easily scan through to see how you can make simple choices to change your eating for the better. Manageable choices that will slowly enable you to bring REAL food into your eating strategy to stay!

Remember, this just gives you an idea what REAL food eating is all about.

BREAKFAST

NO - *Donut*
YES - *Whole Grain Bagel and Peanut Butter*
WHY- Donuts are fried and loaded with bad fat and oodles of sugar. This clogs arteries, gives little to nil nutrition, and sends blood glucose levels temporarily through the roof.

Whole grains made from the whole kernel, provide long-term complex carbohydrate energy with oodles of fiber, vitamin B, and other vital nutrients.

Half a bagel is a serving, and rings in at about 120 calories. A tablespoon of peanut butter offers good fat and protein, with around 100 calories of lasting energy.

NO - *Lucky Charms Cereal*
YES - *Steel Cut Oats*
WHY- Many boxed breakfast cereals are loaded with simple sugars and very little nutrients. Giving you some unstable quick energy that doesn't last.

A 3/4 cup of cooked steel cut oats, has about 150 calories, 25 grams of good carbs, and 4 grams of fiber, with less than 3 grams of fat. You'll also get 7-10 grams of protein according to *LiveStrong*. Which of course helps with cell function, lean muscle building, and fat loss. Iron is also present, which deters fatigue, heart palpitations, headaches and dizziness.

Making your oats with milk adds calcium, to help with energy and skeletal health.

NO- *Sausage*

YES- *Lean Ham*
WHY- Sausage is fatty meat, typically high in bad fat and calories. Lean ham provides the muscle building energizing protein, minus all the saturated fat. Just what your body needs in the morning to get a jumpstart. Have some fresh berries with a little yogurt, or a banana with this, and you've got a fantabulous breakfast!

NO- *Fruit Juices*
YES- *Water*
WHY- Fruit juice is loaded with sugar and very little nutrients. Most have very little actual juice. So you're getting oodles of calories with little nutritional gain.

You can't go wrong with water. There are no calories to worry about, and water in essential for your body to function optimally. At least 6 glasses per day is recommended for the average adult.

NO- *Pop-Tart*
YES- *One Egg and Two Egg-White Omelet*
WHY- One "Cookies and Cream" Pop-Tart has almost 200 calories, where 45 calories are from fat! It has 19 grams of sugar, 35 grams of bad carbs, and just 2 grams of protein. This is according to *Rwservices*.

Eggs on the other hand, are a fantabulous source of protein, and have just 70 calories each. You get iron, vitamin A, D, E, and B12, along with folate, choline, and a few other nutrients. Adding a few extra egg-whites saves some of the fat, and ups the nutrients.

Add a slice of whole grain toast and an orange to this, and you've got one **REAL** way to start your day.

LUNCH

NO- *Bacon and Cheese Panini*
YES- *Whole Grain Chicken Wrap*
WHY- A typical bacon and cheese white Panini can run you around 600 calories and 30 grams of fat! Too many calories and fat, if you're looking to eat **REAL** to lose weight. A whole grain chicken wrap with oodles of veggies and no sauce, has just 150 calories and 5 grams of healthy fat. You can have two and still be miles ahead!

NO- *Plain Bagel with Butter*
YES- *Whole Grain Bagel with Cream Cheese*
WHY- The average store bought plain bagel has 300 calories, according to *Tim Hortons Restaurants.* Add to that almost 50 grams of processed carbs, which delivers short-term energy. One tablespoon of butter is another hundred calories of saturated fat.

The whole grain bagel is just as high in calories, but you're getting complex carbs with fiber, essential minerals, and long-lasting energy. Add some protein and calcium-rich cream cheese in moderation, and you've got a **REAL** healthy lunch!

NO- *Creamy Sun-dried-Tomato Soup*
YES- *Home-made Chicken Noodle Soup*
WHY- Creamy anything screams FAT. This creamy tomato soup is about 230 calories per bowl, with 13 grams of fat. You're better to make your own chicken noodle soup. Back off on the salt, and make sure you add oodles of lean chicken and veggies. You'll get less than half the fat with clear soup, instead of the creamy stuff.

NO- *Chicken Caesar Salad*
YES- *Grilled Chicken Spinach Salad*
WHY- Dressing tends to kill a good thing. Many people easily add 5-6 tablespoons of unhealthy dressing to their salad. That's an extra 600 calories of fat! With the bacon bits and croutons,

you're transforming your "could-be" healthy salad, into an un-healthy mess!

Stick with the salad idea, but go for iron rich spinach, muscle building grilled chicken, and oodles of veggies plate. Eat the salad naked, or have a little dressing on the side if you must. It certainly doesn't hurt to drizzle a little olive-oil based dressing on your healthy meal. Just remember moderation, or you're going to have to put your dreaded fat pants back on again.

NO- *Shepherd's Pie*
YES- *Hearty Chili*
WHY- Most Shepard's Pie is made with pastry, and that's loaded with saturated fat. Think of having a piece of pie with some meat in the middle. You're better option is to get your lean protein with a healthy bowl of home-made chili, loaded with veggies and lean beef, and easy on the salt. In most instances a bowl of **REAL** chili is smarter than a piece of pie!

DINNER

NO- *Fettuccine*
YES- *Whole Wheat Pasta with Chicken*
WHY- Fettuccine is one of those dinners that's comforting. Lots of thick rich creamy sauce, and a whole whack of simple carb white noodles. That's oodles of fat and calories you don't need. Opt for 3/4 up of whole wheat fiber rich pasta with some free-range chicken instead.

NO- *Deep Fried Chicken Wings and Fries*
YES- *Grilled Smoked Salmon with Sweet Potato*
WHY- Deep fried anything is a ticket to run far and fast. You're going to load yourself up with unnecessary saturated fat, simple sugar carbs, and very little nutrients. Keep it real by opting for omega fatty acid rich salmon, and heart healthy good carb sweet potato. This'll give you the learn protein, complex

energy carbs, and vital nutrients your body needs to blast fat and get healthy.

NO- *Baby Back Ribs and Onion Rings*
YES- *Baked Pork Tenderloin*
WHY- It's the sauce on the ribs that kills you! The high sugars and oodles of sodium in one serving, is more than you need the whole day. Add an order of onion rings to the meal, and you're looking at around 2000 calories, and 35 grams of saturated fat!

A 6 ounce serving of pork tenderloin is just 200 calories, 40 grams of protein, and just 3 grams of fat! Add a wallop of steamed veggies to that, and you're going to get a full belly with less than a quarter the calories of the ribs, with **REAL** wholesome food.

SNACKS

NO- *Doritos (30g)*
YES- *Sunflower Seeds (1/4 cup)*
WHY- The chips are processed with no nutrients, and have 10 grams of fat and 40 grams of sugar!

Sunflower seeds have about 160 calories per serving, and give you only 1.5 grams of saturated fat, and 4 grams of fiber. A great pick-me-up that's totally natural.

NO- *Twix Bar*
YES- *Fage 2% Peach Yogurt*
WHY- Chocolate bars are simple sugar foods that spike your blood glucose levels. One bar rings in at almost 300 calories, and has 14 grams of fat, according to *Fitness Magazine.*

This all-natural snack has only 120 calories per serving, with 2.5 grams of fat, 18 grams of good carbs, and over 10 grams of protein!

NO- *Alpen Strawberry & Yogurt Bars*
YES- *Kashi Dark Chocolate Coconut Fruit and Grain Bar*
WHY- These Alpen bars per serving have 120 calories and 3 grams of fat. Problem is, they have almost a third of their weight in sugar. This is NOT healthy for you. Looks healthy and is packaged healthy, but you can do better.

This granola isn't plucked from the earth. But it's made with all-natural ingredients, no preservatives, artificial ingredients, or additives. It's got about 120 calories, 4 grams of fat, 20 grams of healthy carbs, and 4 grams of fiber and protein!

NO- *Chewy Fruit Snacks*
YES- *Stretch Island Fruit Co. Strawberry Pomegranate Sunshine Fruit Leather*
WHY- Fruit snacks are a favorite with kids. Sure they're low in calories, but they've also often got corn syrup, sugar, modified corn starch, citric acid, lactic acid, juice from concentrate, artificial flavor, gelatin, sodium citrate, carnauba wax, and coloring. This is a processed food with ingredients your body doesn't need.

This 15 gram snack is made completely with fruit puree and juice concentrates. And it's got a half serving of fruit with each stick. Not as good as the real deal, but close. Each has about 45 grams of fat, 11 grams of carbs, and a gram of fiber.

NO- *Ritz Mini Cracker Sandwiches*
YES- *Bear Naked Native Mango Agave Almond Granola*
WHY- One serving of these Ritz bits has twice the saturated fat of a whole order of chicken nuggets, according to *MNN Health.* You're looking at over 200 calories, 4 grams of saturated fat, and almost 6 grams of sugar, in a measly 40 gram serving.

This tasty granola treat has no high-fructose corn syrup, and is sweetened naturally with agave nectar glaze. You get whole grain oats, dried mangos, brown rice syrup and honey. 1/4 cup serving is around 140 calories, with 4 grams of good fat, 18 grams of carbs, 3 grams of fiber, and 3 grams of protein.

My Thoughts...

Life is all about choice. And when it comes to figuring out your eating strategy, it's not about being perfect, but making better choices each day towards a healthier more natural you.

There will be times when you're in a pinch and there's really nothing 100% for you to eat. Relax and opt for the next best thing in this situation. Set yourself up for success by planning your meals beforehand, so that you aren't stuck in a pinch and tempted with junky food.

Start learning how to make more natural food choices to better your health. Step by step you will get there, just stick with it!

Chapter Eight - REAL Weight Loss Action Tips

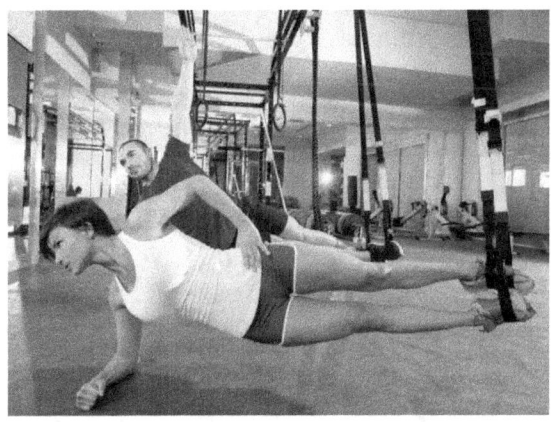

You don't have to go to the extreme to lose weight and get healthy. We've all tried the starvation thing. Or how about not eating anything after 6 pm? There are ten zillion tricks people claim make it easy as pie to lose weight.

Here are a few tactics you can use to lose weight from nutrition and fitness experts. In my books that holds a heck of a lot more credibility than your coffee-table-talk friends!

*NEVER ENTER THE FAMISHED MODE!

If you ignore your hunger long enough, and allow your emotions to call the shots, you'll lose control of your healthy eating and regret it soon after. By taking the time to plan ahead, and always have a few healthy snacks in your purse or bag, you're not going to wind up giving into the vending machine cuz you can't wait till you get home from work to eat.

Snack Ideas...

*Container with 1/4 cup nuts
*Banana
*1/2 whole grain peanut butter sandwich
*Bag of raw veggies
*Whole-fat yogurt with berries
*Box of raisins

*Calculate Your BMI!

You've gotta know how many calories in general your body needs at rest, to maintain your weight. If you know this, you can figure out how you're going to eat real food to maintain your weight, lose weight, or gain it, depending on your circumstance.

The BMI calculator takes your height, weight, sex, and activity level, and roughly computes how many calories your system needs to keep your weight steady. It's definitely a place to start. There are oodles of online calculators your can use, or just ask your doctor or trainer to help you with it.

Know your bottom line so you can set yourself up for success!

*Workout Like You Mean It!

This is one of those things that all comes down to choice. Experts agree, that effort equals reward here. Intense interval training is the most effective route to burn fat quickly, according to *WebMD* experts.
It's where you alternate short periods of intense weight training and cardiovascular activity, with lower effort timed periods, for maximum lean muscle gain and cardiovascular strengthening.

This type of exercise keeps your mind and body guessing, using the maximum calories available. Cross-fit, boot camp sessions, and circuit training, are all awesome intense interval training workouts.

If you're serious about losing weight, you might as well work hard and get there faster. Makes sense don't you think?

The Heart and Stroke Foundation of Canada, recommends at least 30 minutes of intense cardiovascular activity daily, and 15-20 minutes of weight training 2-3 days a week. That's a great place to start!

*Learn To Eat To Lose Weight

If you want to lose weight, you've got to de-program your "starvation" thinking, and program in eating **REAL** healthy food.

According to the *Leslie Bonci*, dietician for the Pittsburgh Steelers, you've gotta eat right to lose weight. If you don't give your body the minimum calories it requires each day to function, it will fight you on weight loss. Your metabolism will grind to a halt, energy levels will drop, and your body will literally try and hoard every carrot stick you eat, trying to protect you from starving.

FACT: When you stop eating, your body interprets that as danger. Intrinsically it slows everything down to conserve energy. It doesn't trust you to feed it enough fuel to run. Learn to fuel your body with real food in the right amounts, and your body will reward you!

*Opt For Red, Orange, and Green

Lean protein and complex carbohydrates are the base of healthy **REAL** food eating to lose weight. To help find balance, think red for muscle building meat, and orange and green for healthy protective antioxidants, and fiber rich carbs. Not to mention the oodles of essential nutrients and long-term energy. This comes from the expert advice in, *The Secret of Skinny: How Salt Makes You Fat.*

*Become a Mini-Meal Eater

Nutritionists from *Calories per Hour*, report there are numerous advantages to eating smaller healthy meals throughout the day, including...

-Decreases the likelihood to overeat
-Levels blood sugars
-Reduces cravings
-Controls mood
-Keeps energy constant
-Increases metabolism

*Drink Up

Experts at *prevention.com*, say you're more likely to get bloated with water by not drinking enough. Drinking at least 6-8 glasses of water per day ensures your body runs optimally. It also gives you that "full" feeling, so you eat less.

*Zone In On Nutrients, NOT Calories

By ensuring you eat adequate lean protein, complex carbs, and good fat, you're more likely to get the right mix of energy, than if you're just looking to have a specific amount of calories. Better **REAL** food delivers longer lasting energy that's nutrient dense, and packs more power per punch.

Less is more when you're paying attention to the macronutrients and micronutrients your body needs.

*Learn Portion Control

You train yourself to expect WAY too much food. You really don't need two chicken breasts for dinner. You eat it because it's there. Step by step learn portion control. Fill your dinner plate with proper portions. If you're still hungry after your chicken breast, small sweet potato, and cup of steamed broccoli, have another cup of broccoli. Or you could opt for a cup of fresh fruit.

The idea is to learn proper portions, eat them, and give yourself time to EXPECT smaller portions. Stick with it and it WILL happen. And you're waist will get smaller too.

*Keep a Food Journal

This is a REALLY tough move to do out of the starting gates. But it will help you realize just how much food you've taught yourself to eat. From there, you can digest this information and start making changes to eat less and expend more energy.

A great way to keep yourself on track and watch your progress!

*Get Support

Change is freakin tough. We are resistant to change and love habit, good or bad. Making sure your family and friends, doctor, trainer, and any other people you depend on know your plans to eat healthier with REAL food and lose weight, will increase the odds you'll make it stick.

Final Thoughts

According to The Atlantic Publication, *medical researchers have found the scientifically proven best diet of all is* **REAL** *food. In other words, there are pluses and minuses for all the eating strategies out there. So there's no one clear winner.*

By taking the time to make sure you're giving your body clean healthy fuel, providing all the energizing macronutrients and system strengthening micronutrients, you'll lose weight and most importantly increase the chances of getting healthy for the long run.

There really is no room for processed foods in healthy living. Problem is, we live in a world centered around convenience. Too far away from the clean eating of our ancient ancestors. Where everything they ate came straight from Mother Nature, straight into the body, with no processing, fats, sugars, salts, or preservatives added.

The Great News!!!

AlterNet *researchers report, science says, you can retrain your brain to actually want healthy REAL food.*

Nutrition and Diabetes *published a study that found you can condition the brain to create new circuits to want healthy food, and skip past the circuits telling you to want toxic processed fast foods.*

Your eating habits are learned, and good or bad, they can be unlearned.

COMMON SENSE ALERT - Science How Stuff Works, *says it takes approximately 30 days of removing a habit to reach the first threshold of breaking it. From there, you've gotta put measures in place to ensure you don't fall back into the habit. So if you quit smoking, it's important you aren't around cigarettes for more than just 30 days. Just cuz you are still vulnerable to the habit.*

Small continuous steps are best. One action at a time, and replace the bad eating habit with a better one. Then rinse and repeat.

The only sure-fire way a habit will stick, is to commit to repeating the action over and over again.

*Keep filling your plate with healthy **REAL** food habits, and those unhealthy old eating habits will soon become ancient history.*

I hope you've enjoyed reading this introductory health and wellness book!

If you've gained just one helpful piece of information from my Real Food Diet masterpiece, then I'm one happy camper!

To your fantabulous health!

Last Thoughts…

*THANK-YOU for reading my masterpiece. I hope you learned a little something, or at least got a few smiles.
*I would appreciate a millisecond or three of your time for a quick review, to help me build my masterful book empire higher.
*Whatever you do, don't forget to smile, and of course, check out my website for more of my e-Book masterpieces at: www.flawlesscreativewriting.com

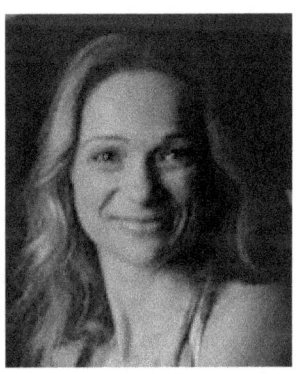

Thank you!
Cathy ☺

www.ingramcontent.com/pod-product-compliance
Lightning Source LLC
Chambersburg PA
CBHW060645290526
45793CB00001B/399